13 Amazing Truths About Pregnancy and Ovulation

Your Roadmap To Successful Conception and Pregnancy

By Kimberley Garcia

Copyright

Kimberley Garcia is the owner of the copyrighted text for the year 2024. The owner retains all rights. Without the prior written permission of the publisher, no portion of this book may be reproduced, stored, or transmitted in any form or by any means, including electronic, mechanical, photocopying, recording, scanning, or any other method.

The only exceptions to this rule are brief quotations that are included in critical reviews and certain other noncommercial uses that are permitted by copyright law.

Disclaimer

The material contained in this book is included solely to provide educational and informational content, and it is not meant to serve as medical advice. Readers are strongly encouraged to discuss their health issues and requirements with registered medical experts who are competent in the field.

The author and publisher of this book do not make any claims or guarantees on the correctness, applicability, suitability, or completeness of the information included within this book. For any loss, injury, or damage that may be experienced directly or indirectly as a result of the use or application of any material included in this book, they expressly disclaim any responsibility for such occurrences. Readers are completely accountable for carrying out their acts and making their own choices.

About The Author

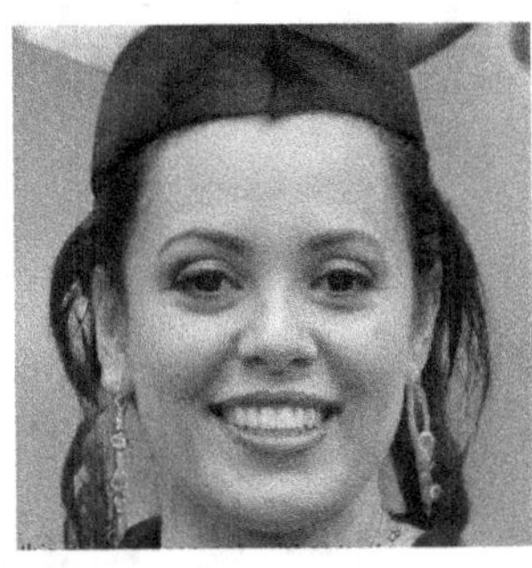

Kimberley Garcia is a fervent supporter of activities that promote the health and well-being of women. The transformational potential of information and empowerment concerning reproductive health is something that she has seen directly as a medical practitioner who is committed to their work and has years of experience in the area.

With a genuine dedication to delivering accurate and accessible information, Kimberley went on a quest to demystify the mysteries of pregnancy and ovulation. Through her work, she strives to enable individuals to make educated decisions about their reproductive journey, whether they are trying to conceive or simply seeking to better understand their bodies.

Beyond her professional accomplishments, Kimberley has a great personal life as a dedicated wife with a family-oriented personality. She believes in the significance of combining business objectives with personal connections and enjoys the moments spent with her loved ones.

In her leisure time, Kimberley likes immersing herself in reading, trying new cuisines, and fostering her creative side through writing. She is truly thankful for the chance to share her expertise and insights with readers via her writing, and she aims to inspire and motivate others on their road to maximum health and happiness.

Table Of Contents

INTRODUCTION

I wrote this book, **13 Amazing Truths About Pregnancy and Ovulation**, to discuss the fascinating subjects of conception, pregnancy, and fertility. If you are considering having a child, striving to get pregnant, or simply fascinated by learning more about how reproduction may work, my comprehensive book will offer you all the most important information and motivation.

Pregnancy and ovulation are important topics that concern millions of people around the world. Unfortunately, various myths and rumors often occur around them. At the same time, the topic of ovulation timing, as well as factors that can affect the ability to conceive, are quite relevant and interesting.

In this book, I look at 13 essential truths about pregnancy and ovulation, which reveal various aspects of this mesmerizing path. I debunk myths, give practical advice, and delve into the latest scientific research to help you confidently and efficiently cope with the difficulties of conception.

As you go through the pages, you will find that becoming pregnant is not always as straightforward as it may look. I cover the variability in ovulation time, the implications of age on fertility, and how lifestyle choices can influence reproductive health. I expose myths connected to contraception and fertility and empower you with the knowledge essential to making informed decisions about your reproductive path.

This book is intended for women attempting to conceive, partners assisting, or anybody interested in learning about pregnancy. It attempts to educate and encourage optimism and confidence along the route to parenting.

So, join me as we go on this informative trip through the astonishing realities surrounding pregnancy and ovulation. Let us empower ourselves with information, accept the complexity of conception, and enjoy the wonder of life in all its grandeur.

When it comes to ovulation and pregnancy, there are a lot of myths and misunderstandings out there. And a lot of the uncertainty is understandable—it is complicated! From how lengthy your period is to when exactly ovulation (and your viable window) happens, it's acceptable if you have some question marks surrounding the whole process. If that's the case, we've got you covered. Read on for a summary of crucial truths and facts regarding ovulation, from fertile age to period sex and beyond.

IT CAN TAKE MULTIPLE MONTHS TO GET PREGNANT

You may have gotten the idea in your high school sex education class that getting pregnant is almost too simple. One time in bed, and that's it—you'll be expecting.

But the fact is that few individuals become pregnant the first month they attempt. It's totally common to wait up to six months to get pregnant. Some expectant parents take up to a year to conceive, and that's also within the scope of normal.

How fast can you expect to get pregnant? After conducting my study, I learned that, after three months of trying, 68% of the couples were pregnant. After a year, 92% conceived. But it's vital to remember that these birthing people were using fertility tracking procedures. The main line is that it's different for everyone, and there is no magic number for how long it takes. That said, if you still haven't conceived after a year of trying (or after six months if you're over 35), it's crucial to reach out to a healthcare practitioner.

Starting the road toward becoming a parent is a thrilling and often long-awaited milestone in the lives of many individuals. However, the process of conceiving a child is not always as quick or straightforward as one may assume. It might take several months to successfully become pregnant.

Understanding the Timing

In plain terms, some people or couples may get pregnant rapidly, within a few tries. However, it's crucial to remember that this isn't the same for everyone. On average, it might take up to six months for a healthy couple who are attempting to conceive. Research suggests that only approximately 30% of couples get pregnant on the first try, whereas the majority conceive within six tries.

Factors Influencing Conception

Numerous variables might impact the time it takes to conceive, including age, overall health, lifestyle factors, and underlying medical issues. For example, growing maternal age can impact fertility, with a progressive drop in fertility reported as women approach their late 30s and early 40s. Similarly, some health disorders, such as polycystic ovarian syndrome (PCOS) or endometriosis, can influence fertility and extend the time it takes to conceive.

Managing Expectations

Trying to get pregnant may be challenging, especially when it comes to dealing with expectations. Many individuals desire a quick and simple road to conception, but it's crucial to be patient and realistic. Knowing that it can take time can decrease the tension and concern that sometimes accompany this procedure. It's also good to discuss this freely with your spouse and obtain assistance from healthcare specialists or support groups while you go through this journey.

Tips for Optimizing Fertility

Even though getting pregnant may not happen right away, there are things that people can do to boost their chances of conceiving. This involves having a healthy lifestyle by eating healthily, exercising, avoiding smoking, limiting alcohol intake, and managing stress. Keeping track of ovulation and having intercourse on the most fertile days of the menstrual cycle might help boost the odds of getting pregnant.

It's crucial to remember that becoming pregnant may take time and patience. By learning the factors that impact conception, having realistic expectations, and actively trying to boost fertility, individuals and couples may approach the process of becoming parents with confidence and strength. It's vital to remember that each pregnancy journey is different, and getting aid and advice during this time may be immensely useful.

OVULATION DOESN'T ALWAYS OCCUR ON DAY 14 OF YOUR CYCLE

Ovulation might take place on the fourteenth day of your cycle. However, it is equally possible that it will not. It is neither unusual nor abnormal to experience ovulation to occur as early as day 6 or day 7 or as late as day 19 or day 20.

During their education on female reproduction, the majority of individuals are instructed that the typical duration of the female cycle is 28 days, and that ovulation takes place at the midpoint on day 14. The phrase "on average" is the catchphrase here. When it comes to fertility, a healthy individual can have a cycle that lasts as little as 21 days or as long as 35 days, and any of these cycles can be deemed to be perfectly normal. The duration of the entire cycle determines whether the day of ovulation occurs earlier or later than that of the previous day.

On the 14th day of a menstrual cycle that lasts for 28 days, many people assume that ovulation takes place. This is a simplified explanation. The fact of the matter is, however, that the time of ovulation is more complicated and varies from person to person. In this chapter, we will go over the specifics of when ovulation takes place, as well as the reasons why it is essential to be aware that it does not always take place in the manner that is anticipated.

Understanding the Menstrual Cycle

Before reviewing the numerous times at which ovulation might occur, let's quickly go over the menstrual cycle. The menstrual cycle is made up of two primary phases: the follicular phase and the luteal phase. In the follicular phase, follicles in the ovaries develop to prepare for ovulation. Around the middle of the cycle, ovulation happens, which is when an egg is released from the ovary. After ovulation, the luteal phase begins, during which the uterus prepares ready for a future pregnancy. If fertilization doesn't happen, menstruation begins, and the cycle starts over again.

Variability in Ovulation Timing

Ovulation, the release of an egg from the ovary, does not usually happen on the 14th day of a woman's menstrual cycle, as many assume. The timing of ovulation can change widely from person to person and even vary from one menstrual cycle to another. Various factors, such as the duration of the menstrual cycle, hormonal changes, stress, sickness, and lifestyle choices, can all impact when ovulation occurs.

Tracking Ovulation

Because ovulation may occur at different times for each individual, it can be difficult to track, but it is crucial, especially for those attempting to get pregnant. Several approaches can assist in anticipating ovulation, such as monitoring basal body temperature, analyzing changes in cervical mucus, utilizing ovulation predictor kits, and keeping track of menstrual cycle trends. By employing one or a combination of these strategies, individuals can better understand their ovulation cycles and boost their chances of conceiving.

Optimizing Conception Timing

Understanding that ovulation doesn't always occur on day 14 of the cycle is vital for maximizing conception timing. Instead of depending on a one-size-fits-all strategy, people should focus on determining their fertile window—the days leading up to and shortly following ovulation—when conception is most likely to occur. By scheduling intercourse deliberately during this fertile window, people might increase their chances of conceiving.

It's vital to note that the timing of ovulation varies substantially from person to person. Ovulation may not always happen on the 14th day of the menstrual cycle, therefore presuming this might result in misunderstandings and missed chances to conceive. By knowing about the subtleties of ovulation timing and adopting accurate ways to detect ovulation, individuals may manage their reproductive health better and maximize their probability of falling pregnant at the most suitable period.

OVULATION CAN HAPPEN FROM EITHER OVARY

Your body does not have a defined pattern of alternating when the ovary releases an egg each month. Ovulation can happen on either side, and it is normal for some people to ovulate more frequently on one side than on the other. This might be either the left or right ovary, depending on numerous conditions. This may be why you feel ovulation discomfort more often on one side than the other.

Ovulation is a key period in the menstrual cycle when a mature egg is released from the ovary, playing a vital part in the process of conception. It's crucial to note that ovulation doesn't simply happen in one ovary; it can occur in either the left or right ovary, and occasionally even in both simultaneously, a condition referred to as bilateral ovulation.

Recognizing this information about ovulation is vital for those wanting to conceive. It underlines the significance of taking into consideration both ovaries while monitoring fertility and establishing the ideal moment for intercourse.

The ovaries are key organs in the reproductive system, placed on either side of the uterus. Each ovary includes follicles that hold immature eggs, which develop during the menstrual cycle under the influence of hormones. Ovulation, where a mature egg is delivered, can occur from either ovary in a given cycle. In certain situations, both ovaries may release eggs concurrently, boosting the odds of pregnancy.

Bilateral ovulation, where eggs are released from both ovaries in the same cycle, is less common yet feasible. This heterogeneity in ovulation underscores the complexity of fertility and the significance of tracking tools to maximize the timing of conception. Understanding the possibility of bilateral ovulation is critical for determining fertility, especially in circumstances where one ovary may be damaged.

Ovulation can come from either ovary or even both at the same time. This highlights how delicate and unexpected the reproductive process may be, stressing the significance of tailored techniques for tracking fertility and trying to conceive. By being informed of the likelihood of ovulation from either side, individuals may take proactive actions to boost their chances of getting pregnant and start their route to becoming parents with certainty.

YES, YOU CAN GET PREGNANT DURING YOUR PERIOD

Contrary to what most people believe, beginning menstruation does not necessarily indicate that it is a "safe" time to avoid becoming pregnant. Under some conditions, you can become pregnant when you are on your period.

Some individuals are under the incorrect impression that if they are still experiencing their period, they are not yet in the "fertile window." (This refers to the five to six days that a woman has during her cycle during which she has the potential to get pregnant.) It is possible to conceive through sexual activity during your period if your cycle is short and you ovulate on day 7 or day 8 of your cycle.

Dispelling Myths

Many individuals are under the incorrect impression that a woman cannot become pregnant if she is experiencing menstruation.

This view, on the other hand, disregards the reality that menstrual cycles don't always follow the same pattern and that sperm might remain in the female body for several days. Although there is a lesser likelihood of becoming pregnant during menstruation compared to other periods in the menstrual cycle, it is still possible to become pregnant during menstruation.

Understanding The Fertility Window

To have a better understanding of the likelihood of becoming pregnant when one is experiencing menstruation, it is essential to be aware of the reproductive window. The interval of time during a woman's menstrual cycle during which the likelihood of conceiving a child is at its highest is referred to as the fertility window. This window normally covers the days before and after ovulation, but the exact date might change for each person.

Factors Influencing Fertility During Menstruation:

- Short Menstrual Cycles: Women with shorter menstrual cycles may ovulate soon after their period finishes, which might enhance the odds of falling pregnant during their period.

- Prolonged Sperm Survival: Sperm can survive in the female reproductive canal for several days, particularly in optimum conditions. If intercourse happens around the end of menstruation and sperm stays viable until ovulation, pregnancy can occur.
- Irregular Menstrual Cycles: Irregular menstrual cycles might make it tough to estimate ovulation effectively. In such instances, conception during menstruation becomes a possibility, especially if ovulation happens earlier or later than predicted.

Practical Considerations

While the possibility of conception during menstruation is quite low, it's vital to examine the practical consequences

- Use of contraceptives: If avoiding pregnancy is a priority, using dependable contraceptive techniques regularly and appropriately is vital, regardless of the menstrual cycle phase.
- Tracking Menstrual Cycles: Monitoring menstrual cycles and detecting patterns of

ovulation can help individuals make educated decisions regarding their fertility and contraceptive options.

While conception during menstruation is less common, it is not impossible. Understanding the variables impacting fertility during the menstrual cycle is vital for making educated decisions regarding reproductive health and contraception. By refuting myths and embracing facts, individuals may manage their reproductive journey with confidence and empowerment.

IF YOU'RE TRYING TO CONCEIVE: HAVE SEX BEFORE YOU OVULATE

When it comes to trying to conceive, timing is important. Many couples wrongly assume that having intercourse right after ovulation is the most efficient method to get pregnant. However, the fact is exactly the reverse.

At first glance, it appears to make sense that the egg has to be present before you put in the sperm. However, that's not how it works.

First of all, sperm may survive in the female reproductive system for up to six days. The sperm will die off as the days pass, so the closer to ovulation you have intercourse, the better. But they don't need to get there "at the moment" of ovulation.

Secondly, and maybe most crucially, the egg becomes nonviable very rapidly. If a sperm cell doesn't fertilize the egg within 12 to 24 hours of being discharged from the ovary, pregnancy can't occur. That doesn't imply you shouldn't have sex after ovulation either; just that pre-ovulation intercourse might enhance your chances of pregnancy.

The Importance of Pre-Ovulation Intercourse

Having intercourse before ovulation implies that there will already be sperm in the fallopian tubes when the egg is released. This makes it more possible for the sperm to meet the egg and for fertilization to happen. If you wait until after ovulation to have sex, you can miss this vital moment, which might limit your chances of getting pregnant.

Predicting Ovulation

Predicting when ovulation happens can be challenging, but there are numerous strategies you can apply to identify when you are most fertile. These strategies include keeping track of your menstrual cycle, noticing changes in cervical mucus, and employing ovulation prediction kits. By monitoring these signs, you may optimize the time of intercourse to correspond with your most fertile phase, boosting the odds of conception.

Tips for Maximizing Conception Success

To enhance your chances of conception, try the following tips:

- Track Your Menstrual Cycle: Keep a diary of your menstrual cycles to find patterns and forecast ovulation.
- Monitor Cervical Mucus: Pay attention to variations in cervical mucus consistency and texture, since they might suggest when you're most fertile.
- Use Ovulation Predictor Kits: Ovulation prediction kits detect the spike in luteinizing hormone (LH) that happens right before ovulation, letting you determine your fertile days.
- Have Regular Intercourse: Aim to have intercourse every 1-2 days within your reproductive window to ensure sperm are there when ovulation happens.
- Prioritize Relaxation: Stress can impair fertility, so prioritize relaxation activities such

as meditation, yoga, or deep breathing exercises.

By following these suggestions and acknowledging the significance of having intercourse before ovulation, you may boost your chances of becoming pregnant and start your road to becoming a parent with confidence. Remember, being patient and persistent is key, and it is crucial to take care of oneself both physically and mentally at this time.

HAVING SEX EVERY DAY WON'T NECESSARILY MAKE YOU GET PREGNANT QUICKER

Having sex every day may not necessarily boost your chances of becoming pregnant faster. While it is feasible to have sex daily if wanted, there is no evidence to suggest that it enhances fertility. Frequent intercourse might lead to weariness and dissatisfaction, especially if pregnancy does not occur in the first month.

The key to conception is not the number of sexes but rather timing them appropriately, such as having intercourse every few days or during your most fertile days. Even if you have sex three times a week, you are likely to hit your most fertile moment. Conception is regulated by several physiological aspects beyond merely time, so just having more sex does not ensure a speedy pregnancy. If time were the sole determinant, more people would conceive in the first month of trying.

Sperm Health and Quantity

Contrary to common perception, having intercourse every day may not necessarily be advantageous for conception, particularly if it leads to a decline in sperm quality or quantity. While frequent ejaculation is typically regarded as healthy for males, it's vital to provide an appropriate recovery period for sperm generation between ejaculations.

Studies show that ejaculating every day might lead to a decreased sperm count and slower sperm motility, both of which are required for successful conception. Furthermore, frequent ejaculation may also diminish the concentration of seminal fluid, which is vital for nourishing and preserving sperm.

Finding the Right Balance

Instead of merely having sex more often while attempting to get pregnant, couples should focus on having intercourse during the most fertile days of the woman's menstrual cycle. In this manner, they can boost their chances of conceiving without affecting the quality of the man's sperm.

It's also crucial to understand that stress and anxiety can influence a couple's desire for sex and intimacy, which might make it difficult to get pregnant. It's crucial to establish a balance between deliberately scheduling intercourse and keeping a calm and comfortable attitude toward intimacy.

Having sex during the fertile window is vital for getting pregnant, but having sex every day might not make it happen faster. It's crucial to understand the menstrual cycle, have intercourse at the proper time, and maintain healthy sperm health. By striking a balance and keeping patient and relaxed, couples can boost their chances of beginning a family.

THE SIGNS OF OVULATION AREN'T ALWAYS OBVIOUS

There are various techniques you may use to track or try to identify ovulation, including monitoring your basal body temperature, detecting changes in cervical mucus, utilizing ovulation predictor tests, and more. Some people find one or a combination of these strategies to be successful and have no problem implementing them.

For some people, using a basal body temperature chart to track ovulation may not be successful. This might be owing to having a convoluted sleep routine or trouble remembering to consistently take and record their temperature every morning. Additionally, some individuals may struggle to identify variations in their cervical mucus from week to week. Even ovulation test kits, which are regarded to be accurate, might be tricky to interpret. It is not always straightforward to establish if the test line is darker than the control line.

If you are anxious about not experiencing indicators of ovulation, it may be useful to consult with a healthcare specialist. It is conceivable that you are having problems recognizing ovulation because you are not ovulating consistently or at all. Ovulation difficulties, such as anovulation, might be a potential explanation for female infertility.

Common Signs of Ovulation

Some people may have apparent signs of ovulation, such as stomach pain or changes in cervical mucus, while others may have more modest clues or no symptoms at all. Common indicators of ovulation include:

- Changes in cervical mucus: As ovulation approaches, cervical mucus may become clear, slick, and stretchy, matching the nature of egg whites. This fertile cervical mucus assists in promoting sperm movement and raises the chance of pregnancy.
- Basal body temperature (BBT) changes: Following ovulation, a woman's basal body temperature normally rises somewhat due to an increase in progesterone levels. Tracking BBT can help pinpoint the date of ovulation retrospectively, but it is not predictive of future ovulation.

- Ovulation pain or mittelschmerz: Some people may suffer slight stomach discomfort or pain, known as mittelschmerz, around the time of ovulation. This discomfort is assumed to originate from the ejection of the egg from the ovary and is typically short-lived.
- Increased libido: Hormonal changes related to ovulation can contribute to an increase in sexual desire for certain individuals, functioning as a natural indicator of fertility.

Variability in Ovulation Signs

It is vital to note that the signs of ovulation can change from one individual to another and can also vary from one menstrual cycle to another. Some people may have frequent and immediately detectable symptoms, while others may suffer shifts or may not have any obvious indicators at all. Furthermore, variables like stress, sickness, or hormone imbalances might impact the occurrence and intensity of ovulation symptoms.

Although the signals of ovulation might be different for each individual and not always simple to spot, having a clear grasp of how ovulation occurs and adopting monitoring tools can help people take control of their reproductive health. By paying attention to subtle indications and collaborating with healthcare specialists, individuals can boost their chances of getting pregnant and fulfilling their family planning objectives.

OVULATION IS ONLY ONE ELEMENT OF GETTING PREGNANT

Ovulation is necessary for getting pregnant, as it involves the release of an egg from the ovary. However, simply having an egg is not enough to conceive a child. The egg must be able to travel through the fallopian tubes to reach the uterus. If the fallopian tubes are blocked or if there are problems with the partner's sperm, then pregnancy may not be possible. In other words, both the egg and the pathway to the egg must be functioning properly for conception to occur.

Infertility can be present without clear symptoms, and sometimes the cause remains unknown. Some fertility issues may not be evident without specific tests. For instance, the fertility of a partner's sperm or the condition of a person's fallopian tubes may require lab testing for an accurate assessment. Ovulation, while important, is just one aspect of the complex picture of fertility.

The Role of Sperm

One key aspect in the process of conception is the existence of healthy sperm. Without healthy sperm, fertilization cannot take place. Sperm must pass via the cervix, uterus, and fallopian tubes to reach the egg. It is vital to determine the health, count, motility (movement), and morphology of sperm to enhance conception.

The Importance of Cervical Mucus

Cervical mucus is vital for conception because it generates a suitable environment for sperm to move through the female reproductive system. The texture and quality of cervical mucus alter during the menstrual cycle, becoming more supportive of sperm survival and motility around the time of ovulation.

The Uterine Environment

After fertilization, the fertilized egg has to attach itself to the uterine lining to start a pregnancy. The state of the uterus, which is impacted by hormonal fluctuations and the general health of the reproductive system, is vital for the successful implantation of the egg.

Hormonal Balance

Hormones are vital for managing the menstrual cycle and assisting with ovulation. When hormone levels are not balanced, it can impact fertility, which can be caused by illnesses like polycystic ovarian syndrome (PCOS) or thyroid issues. It is crucial to diagnose and address hormonal abnormalities in order to increase fertility.

Lifestyle Factors

In addition to biological variables, the decisions we make in our everyday lives can also impact our capacity to conceive a child. Things like what we eat, how often we exercise, how stressed we are, and our exposure to certain environmental conditions can all have a role in our reproductive health and fertility. By making good lifestyle choices, including eating a balanced diet, being active, managing stress, and avoiding hazardous substances, we can boost our chances of getting pregnant and having a successful pregnancy.

Medical Interventions

Some people may need medical intervention to handle reproductive concerns. Assisted reproductive technologies like in vitro fertilization (IVF) or intrauterine insemination (IUI) can aid people and couples in becoming pregnant when natural conception is not effective.

Ovulation is vital for getting pregnant, but it is just one element of the whole process. By understanding and addressing diverse variables that impact fertility and conception, individuals may take control of their reproductive health. This may involve regulating hormones, adopting good lifestyle choices, and getting medical care when necessary. By making proactive efforts, people can boost their odds of becoming parents.

FERTILITY DECLINES AFTER AGE 35, BUT YOU CAN GET PREGNANT AFTER 40

Regardless of how healthy a person is, their capacity to conceive reduces as they age. The odds of getting pregnant at the age of 40 are decreased compared to when they are 30. Female fertility starts to diminish considerably around the age of 35. Due to this drop, it is suggested by specialists that people over the age of 35 who are attempting to conceive should seek assistance for getting pregnant earlier than younger ones.

All being said, it is still possible to get pregnant after the age of 40. Many ladies have successfully given birth to healthy infants, even at the age of 40 or 41. However, the risks of having fertility troubles, miscarriages, and other pregnancy concerns increase once you approach 40. It can also take more time for you to conceive. Despite these dangers, it is vital to remember that being 40 years old does not imply you cannot have a safe pregnancy.

Factors Influencing Fertility After 40

Although age is a significant element in a person's capacity to have children, it is not the only thing that influences their fertility as they become older. Other factors, like as their overall health, lifestyle choices, any medical disorders they may have, and whether they have access to fertility medications, all play a part in determining their ability to conceive after the age of 40. By taking care of these variables and making sensible decisions, people can boost their chances of getting pregnant later in life.

Fertility Options for Individuals Over 40

For those over 40 who are failing to conceive naturally, there are different reproductive alternatives available to satisfy their desire for parenting. These alternatives include assisted reproductive technologies, including in vitro fertilization (IVF), egg donation, and fertility preservation. Individuals in this position should seek counsel from a fertility professional who can make individualized treatment choices based on their unique requirements and circumstances to help them accomplish their goal of becoming parents.

Age is simply one issue to consider when thinking about fertility. Although fertility normally diminishes with age, people over 40 can still achieve their ambition to become parents by making well-informed decisions, employing fertility treatments, and having the support of healthcare experts and loved ones. By being open to numerous alternatives and being strong in tough times, individuals may boldly and resolutely start the route to parenting, no matter how old they are.

MALE FERTILITY ALSO DECLINES WITH AGE

You may have heard of male celebrities having children when they are older than 60 years old. This could make you assume that males can continue to father children at any age, but that is not correct. While men do not undergo a physiologic process like menopause that marks the end of their reproductive years, male fertility does drop as men get older.

When males over the age of 40 father children, there are possible dangers linked to the pregnancy and health of the child. These dangers include a greater possibility of infertility, miscarriage, and stillbirth, as well as an increased risk of certain illnesses and disorders such as autism, bipolar disorder, schizophrenia, and childhood leukemia.

Factors Contributing to Declining Male Fertility

Several factors contribute to the loss of male fertility with age. These include hormonal changes, increased oxidative stress, lifestyle variables such as smoking and excessive alcohol intake, environmental exposures, and underlying medical disorders. While the pace of decline differs across people, men need to be aware of these issues and make proactive efforts to maintain their reproductive health.

Impact on Conception and Pregnancy

The reduction in male fertility with age might have substantial ramifications for couples seeking to conceive. As sperm quality drops, the odds of obtaining a pregnancy may decrease, and the time to conception may be prolonged. Additionally, older paternal age has been connected with an increased risk of various pregnancy difficulties, such as miscarriage, birth deformities, and neurodevelopmental impairments in kids.

Supporting Male Reproductive Health

Maintaining good reproductive health is vital for men of all ages. Adopting a healthy lifestyle, including regular exercise, a balanced diet, appropriate sleep, and stress management, can help boost overall well-being and fertility. Avoiding exposure to environmental contaminants, reducing alcohol intake and smoking, and practicing safe sex are other critical factors in sustaining male reproductive health.

Male fertility changes with age, and knowing these changes is crucial for people and couples beginning on the road to conception and motherhood. By being proactive about reproductive health and getting appropriate medical care when required, men may take positive measures toward conserving and maximizing their fertility, eventually contributing to their general well-being and the achievement of their reproductive aspirations.

BIRTH CONTROL DOES NOT CAUSE INFERTILITY

The worry of infertility is a prevalent issue among people contemplating or utilizing birth control techniques. Many myths and misconceptions surround the issue, leading to undue tension and confusion. In this chapter, we will investigate the facts behind the idea that birth control causes infertility and refute common fallacies related to contraceptive use.

Myth: Birth control causes long-term infertility

Fact: One of the most common fallacies regarding birth control is the assumption that it might lead to irreversible infertility. This myth generally originates from misconceptions about how birth control techniques function and their impact on the body.

Understanding Birth Control Methods

To address this myth, it's vital to understand the various methods of birth control and how they act. Hormonal contraceptives, such as birth control pills, patches, injections, and hormonal intrauterine devices (IUDs), function by adjusting hormone levels to prevent ovulation or conception. Non-hormonal measures, such as barrier methods like condoms and diaphragms, prevent pregnancy by physically stopping sperm from accessing the egg.

Temporary Effects

While certain birth control techniques may briefly decrease fertility after quitting, these effects are often reversible. Hormonal contraceptives may temporarily postpone ovulation and menstrual periods, although fertility normally recovers once the technique is discontinued. Non-hormonal techniques do not interfere with ovulation or hormonal balance and have no long-term influence on fertility.

Fertility After Discontinuation

Numerous studies have demonstrated that the great majority of individuals restore fertility immediately after discontinuing birth control. For most women, menstrual periods return to normal within a few months, and pregnancy becomes feasible. In reality, many individuals conceive immediately after quitting birth control, typically without encountering any problems.

Addressing Concerns

Despite the overwhelming evidence dispelling the myth of birth control-induced infertility, anxieties continue among certain individuals. Healthcare practitioners must address these issues and give factual information to reduce worries and misconceptions. Open communication and education are crucial to allowing individuals to make educated decisions regarding contraception and their reproductive health.

Birth contraception does not cause infertility. While some transitory impacts on fertility may occur with contraceptive usage, the great majority of people restore fertility immediately after cessation.

Understanding how birth control techniques operate and their impact on fertility can help debunk misunderstandings and soothe anxieties. By providing accurate information and promoting open conversation, we can enable individuals to make confident decisions regarding contraception and their reproductive health.

ANY SEXUAL POSITION CAN RESULT IN PREGNANCY

When it comes to conception, one of the most widespread myths is the assumption that various sexual positions enhance or decrease the probability of pregnancy. This chapter tries to refute this misconception and offer clarification on the significance of sexual postures in the conception process.

Dispelling Myths

Many fallacies persist surrounding sexual positions and their claimed influence on fertility. Some feel that particular postures, such as the missionary position, are more favorable to conception, while others say that unusual positions, such as standing or sitting, may impede fertility. However, there is no scientific evidence to back these statements.

Understanding the Physiology

In truth, the position in which intercourse occurs has negligible influence on the chance of pregnancy. The important step in conception is the effective transport of sperm into the female reproductive system, where they may travel to meet the egg. This procedure can occur regardless of the sexual position.

Factors Affecting Fertility

Instead of focusing on sexual positions, couples seeking to conceive should prioritize aspects that have a bigger influence on fertility, such as scheduling intercourse to coincide with ovulation, keeping a healthy lifestyle, and addressing any underlying medical concerns that may impair conception.

Enjoying Intimacy

Rather than obsessing over the "right" sexual position for conception, couples are urged to focus on enjoying intimacy and connecting emotionally with their spouse. Healthy, happy relationships are a crucial part of general well-being and can significantly improve fertility.

Tips for Couples

- Communicate freely with your spouse about your wants, worries, and expectations around conception.
- Prioritize closeness and emotional connection in your relationship, since this can increase fertility and general well-being.
- Remember that there is no one-size-fits-all strategy to conception, and what works for one couple may not work for another.
- Consult with a healthcare practitioner if you have been trying to conceive for a lengthy period without success, since there may be underlying reasons leading to infertility.

The assumption that specific sexual positions enhance or reduce the probability of pregnancy is a myth. Any sexual position can result in pregnancy as long as sperm is correctly placed in the female reproductive system. Couples are urged to focus on enjoying intimacy and emphasizing elements that have a bigger influence on fertility, rather than stressing about the "right" sexual position for conception.

THE BOTTOM LINE

As we approach the last chapter of "13 Amazing Truths About Pregnancy and Ovulation," it's time to simplify the abundance of material we've covered into actionable insights and important takeaways. In this last chapter, we review the main facts and give suggestions on how to apply them to your path toward conception and family.

1. Understanding Your Menstrual Cycle:
   - Take the time to understand about your menstrual cycle and how it connects to ovulation.
   - Track your cycle using apps, calendars, or other means to find patterns and forecast fertile days.
2. Timing Intercourse:
   - Recognize that timing intercourse correctly can dramatically boost your chances of conception.
   - Aim to have intercourse in the days preceding ovulation to increase sperm availability when the egg is released.
3. Optimizing Fertility:

- Prioritize your entire health and well-being, since factors like food, exercise, and stress can affect fertility.
- Consider lifestyle improvements and seek help from healthcare specialists if needed to resolve any fertility difficulties.

4. Managing Expectations:
   - Understand that getting pregnant may take time, and it's normal for conception to not happen quickly.
   - Stay patient and cheerful, concentrating on the journey rather than fixating entirely on the ultimate goal of pregnancy.

5. Communicating with Your Spouse:
   - Maintain open and honest communication with your spouse during the conception process.
   - Share your thoughts, concerns, and goals for the future, and work together as a team to manage any problems that occur.

6. Seeking Help:
   - Don't hesitate to seek help from friends, family, or support groups if

you're feeling overwhelmed or uncertain.

- Reach out to healthcare specialists for information and support tailored to your unique requirements and circumstances.

7. Embracing the Journey:
    - Remember that the parenting path is a unique and intensely personal experience for each individual and couple.
    - Embrace the ups and downs, embrace the times of connection and intimacy, and believe in the timing of your fertility journey.

"13 Amazing Truths About Pregnancy and Ovulation" has been developed to empower you with knowledge, debunk myths, and give practical direction as you navigate the wonderful path of conception and motherhood.

May you embrace this journey with confidence, optimism, and a great appreciation for the marvelous process of bringing new life into the world.

Congratulations on taking the initial steps towards forming the family of your dreams. I wish you health, happiness, and countless blessings on your journey to fatherhood.

I HAVE A REQUEST

Dear **Reader**,

I hope this message finds you well. I am writing to kindly request your feedback and review of my recently published book, **"13 Amazing Truths About Pregnancy and Ovulation."** Your thoughts and opinions are incredibly important to me, and I would greatly appreciate your honest review.

Your review will not only provide valuable insights but also help other potential readers make informed decisions about whether to explore the book. As a fellow reader, your perspective is highly regarded.

Here's how you can help:

- *Read the Book*: If you haven't already had the chance to read "[Book Title]," I'd be happy to provide you with a complimentary copy in your preferred format (eBook or paperback).
- *Share Your Review*: After reading the book, please take a moment to share your thoughts by leaving a review on popular book retail

platforms, such as Amazon, Goodreads, or any other platform where you prefer to review books.

- *Be Honest and Constructive*: Your honest opinion is what matters most. Whether you loved the book or had some critical feedback, I welcome your insights. Constructive criticism is just as valuable as praise.
- *Spread the Word*: If you found the book enjoyable and enlightening, consider sharing your review with your friends and family or on your social media platforms to help others discover it.

Your support in providing a review will not only be deeply appreciated, but will also be instrumental in spreading the message and impact of the book. Your input will guide future readers and play a vital role in its success.

Thank you for taking the time to consider my request. Your support means a great deal to me, and I am grateful for your willingness to share your thoughts on **"13 Amazing Truths About Pregnancy and Ovulation."**

I wish you an enriching reading experience, and I look forward to hearing from you.

Warm regards,

Kimberley Garcia

ADDITIONAL RESOURCES

Dear Reader, I am here again:

Thank you for your support and interest in my book, **"13 Amazing Truths About Pregnancy and Ovulation."** If you enjoyed this book and are looking for more valuable resources and engaging content, I would recommend some of my books that you might find intriguing:

1. **"Best Parenting Book For Kids With ADHD"**: *An ADHD Parenting Guide for Raising Hyperactive Kids, Dealing with Behavioral Issues, and Supporting Explosive Children*
2. **"Finding Relief"**: *10 Home Remedies To Relieve Menstrual Cramps*
3. **"Successful Parenting Of Kids With Autism"**: *Easy Steps To Raising Brilliant Autistic Kids*
4. **"Single Mom's Pregnancy Guide"**: *A Comprehensive Guide For Single Mothers*
5. **"Pregnancy Cookbook With Nutritional Information"**: *The Complete Healthy Guide*

To Optimal Prenatal Nutrition And Real Food For Pregnancy With 30+ Recipes For Your Pregnancy Meal Plan

6. **"The Complete Guide For Trending Baby Names In 2024":** *A Thoughtful Up-To-Date Guide To Selecting Unique And Timeless Baby Names For Expecting Mothers, Fathers And Parents*

7. **"Easiest Way To Get Rid Of Pregnancy Hemorrhoids In 2024":** *Your Essential Handbook For Overcoming Pregnancy Hemorrhoids With Confidence*

To explore these books, please visit my Author Central Page on Amazon. **You can scan the QR code below or click the link to visit my Author Central:**

https://www.amazon.com/author/kimberley_garcia

Your continued support means the world to me, and I am committed to providing you with valuable information and inspiration on your journey as a woman.

Thank you for being a part of this community, and I hope my books continue to bring you joy and empowerment.

Warm regards,
Kimberley Garcia

PS: *Don't forget to check out my Author Central page on Amazon to discover more of my books. Your feedback and reviews are always appreciated!*

www.ingramcontent.com/pod-product-compliance
Lightning Source LLC
Chambersburg PA
CBHW051653250726
48653CB00007B/2634